Knock-*knock*

OWEN LEWIS

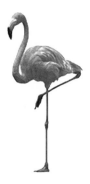

DOS MADRES

2024

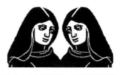

DOS MADRES PRESS INC.

P.O. Box 294, Loveland, Ohio 45140
www.dosmadres.com   editor@dosmadres.com

Dos Madres is dedicated to the belief that the small press is essential to the vitality of contemporary literature as a carrier of the new voice, as well as the older, sometimes forgotten voices of the past. And in an ever more virtual world, to the creation of fine books pleasing to the eye and hand.

Dos Madres is named in honor of Vera Murphy and Libbie Hughes, the "Dos Madres" whose contributions have made this press possible.

Dos Madres Press, Inc. is an Ohio Not For Profit Corporation and a 501 (c) (3) qualified public charity. Contributions are tax deductible.

Executive Editor: Robert J. Murphy

Illustration & Book Design: Elizabeth H. Murphy
www.illusionstudios.net

Typeset in Adobe Garamond Pro & TaxType
ISBN 978-1-962847-01-8
Library of Congress Control Number: 2024930721

GRATITUDE

Special thanks to physician/writer/friends Robert Abrams, Richard Berlin, and Michael Salcman for invaluable suggestions; to Kate Daniels and her pitch-perfect ear; to Fran Quinn, ever the patient and persistent teacher; to the Departments of Geriatric Medicine and Palliative Care Grand Rounds, Weill Cornell Medical Center, where an early version was presented; to Robert Murphy and Elizabeth Murphy, heart, soul, and muscle of Dos Madres Press; and to my wife, Susan, for her love and support of my imaginative explorations.

for Oscar Lifshitz, my namesake

TABLE OF CONTENTS

Knock, knock! Who's there, in the other devil's name?
Faith, here's an equivocator . . .

O, come in, equivocator.

William Shakespeare, *Macbeth*

Knock-*knock*

Prelude: How I Started to Use a Cane

A day of almost rain
I took my umbrella
to be prepared.

It had an oak curved handle
that fitted my palm.
I hadn't noticed at first,

the tap of the wooden end
on the street
just ahead of my right foot.

The motion, a natural
swing forward just ahead
of my right leg, sweet, easy—

I was talking on the phone,
walking steadier, noticed the tap,
and after, the tap-step, a light

knock, a knock like someone's
at the door come to visit,
like company's always arriving

and I feel this step in my hand
and hear it keeping a nice beat.
If my feet are sock-swaddled

they get muffled and vague
and make a kind of shuffle-step,
shuffle-glide, instead of the steady

tap, the tap-step's sure contact
with concrete. Some days I set out,
I'm half-way to downtown, and

I forget. All the names and numbers
are in the phone, I know, but when
the name goes blank, the phone

directory is no use, no use at all.
The tap-step's the only sure thing,
even as my daughter's name

my very own first-born's name
slips my mind and I almost slip
from the sudden blank shock of it,

comes the tap, the tap-step, the tap-
step keeps my feet perfectly in place,
my mind can be anywhere at all.

I haven't imagined I've lost my scarf

then a coat, my phone, the book I am reading.
The ivory cat isn't seen, and I imagine him lost
several hours ago. (Later he appears on my
pillow.)

In my albums
friends and family don't have extra lives.
I make sure
to write their names I'm
trying to remember
the title of the book I look under
the cushions and a stack of journals.

I've got no use for news about news.
No headlines about the scarf or the coat.
Where'd they go?
                    Lost-and-Found
                    is not a planned
                    destination.

When I'm not losing things

they often slip out of my hands.
Before it took itself away,
that book, a tale of a walk along the sea,

   (about love, the best are, about a young
   couple's near misses. Love, a near miss.
   Oh, I am missing   so much)   it

just dropped from my hands, its spine into
my big toe—alarm clock knock of pain, wake,
up—and the cup I held,   as if the handle
had broken off, my hand just forgot how
to keep a grip.   Splash of
               hot   meat
                   broth.
                            Imagine . . .

things often fall with a clatter and break,
but sometimes without a crash or clamor
they pass into another realm, quiet winter-
light draining the day.
                    Then I understand
they're not lost.
                They've moved ahead
without so much as a knock. A prep-team
is stocking up the next time zone.

Like tropical time. Always summer there.
I'll find many things in my little cottage.
More light there. More time   there.
I wonder what time it is in the Care Home.

There they say I might need more care.
There.

I ask my doctor how one can remember

not remembering. He's one of the good ones,
holds my x-rays up to the window. *Hmmm.*
I can see through that. There's a tree bough
growing right across my lungs. In my knees,
a bird nest, my shoulder of garden perennials.
From the MRI, I see a cloud inside my skull.
He's asking about my aches—
I live with them.   What does he do with his?

> (My daughter glares. She comes with that nervous
> cough of hers that always makes me forget what,
> what I want to ask. I should have made a list.)

What about that cumulus? *What about sleep?*
he insists. I insist. What about that cloud?
Am I   a cloud? An i-cloud? Blessèd heavens!

> (They ask me to step outside the office. Listening at
> the door. She's telling the doctor things like I'm a
> misbehaving kid and he's the bow-tied principal.)

He shows me the ventricle, traces a gaping hole.
I won't look.   In it   a mix of all the words
I can't remember, tumbling around. The letters link
arm in arm   something I'll need to know.   *Next!*

Next! Next! Next!

> (Next is detention in an old age home. What if
> I refuse? What if I get in my car and drive to
> Florida myself? Or Alaska! He calls it a *fugue state*.)

I tell him,

"I, too, am a doctor . . ."

"*Were*, my friend. Were. Your daughter will. . ."

"Will what ? . . "

"What needs to be done."

"I am not,   I am . . .

I had a white coat
with a name stitched
in red script letters
above the pocket . . .

Card carrying

member of the A.M.A. it's always
in my wallet what the letters mean
I don't matter it doesn't matter—
smart and well-educated doctors
can have whole conversations in
quick letter codes—check the CBC,
the U/A, the EEG, ECG, CPK,
they love those lipids, they love ratios,
the BUN/Creatinine, LDL/HDL and

mostly they love to insist—Echo him—
doctor's orders—Echo him!

Marvelous to hear human echoes
and decipher everything hearts say
I take off my shirt and under-shirt
but not my pants the technician
focuses the machine over the knock
deep in my right ventricle and they
seance around my chest and close
their eyes to listen to the knock-
knocking I know the moment

they can hear a first love's echo
and their faces become   beatific!

Get Hold of Yourself:
What You Remember is True

I tell myself to remember my daughter
said we bought the semi-detached cottage
as is and I'm "as is", *caveat emptor.* Buyer
beware. It's decorated in tropical colors
and rattan furniture that creaks louder
than my knees. When I was eight

uncle and aunt and cousins took me
along, we drove three days to Florida,
and this is true, we pulled into a pseudo-
Mexicana "South of the Border" joint,
a welcoming elephant chained to a palm.
Aunt said, "Close the windows!"

Elephant knocked so I opened mine.
He ran his trunk in, across our noses.
Aunt beat his trunk with newspaper
and I kept thinking that elephant
could pick up the whole car or roll
us right off the road or stomp us flat.

We went into the restaurant and since
we were south of the border, probably
Carolina, a sign above the door read
"Whites Only" and my uncle said just
ignore it and one day it will change
and good thing we live up North.

It seems just last month we were
singing *We Shall Overcome* one day
and that's how fast time is and
isn't when change is needed more
than ever.
   I don't know where to
live when change is more than ever.

Knock-

Who's there?

You?

You-who?

You don't even know?

Know what?

You're already in.

In what?

In what, he asks.
Is he still a doctor?

He is, I suppose.

Then he should know.

Know what? Be what? In what?
Until what?

Until . . .

Before my daughter leaves

she always promises she'll be back
in a few days or a few months
and she pocket-pins my name tag
on my shirt and says always wear it
don't take it off and she says *Don't
Worry* and tells me she feels bad
since there's no piano here but
my fingers don't play it anymore
she says just hum the fugue song
but I'm only one voice we need
at least three others she says just
say *Hi* each time the attendant
comes by and start with him but
I know she's even more worried
I'll forget my name lose the tag
so I don't take it off and I'm good
and even when I send the shirt
to the washers they don't take it off
and every day I sit in the sun
a red bench under a blousy date palm
a very friendly lady keeps coming by
and one day she sits on the bench
right next to me and I then realize
it's not a coconut palm but a date
palm and boy am I a dummy and
she asks what my name is I point
to the tag but my name's already
a blue streak and I say that's who
she points to hers laughs so much
there isn't even a smear left on hers
and we become good friends.

Lesson # 13, from the Care Home

Standing on one foot—
an interesting proposition.

It's a balance exercise
my P/T has me do. And

a king once asked a Rabbi
(must have been Hillel)

to explain the whole Torah
standing on one foot he said:

love your neighbor—
he was on   one foot—

and the rest, commentary.
Did he mean actual love

on one foot?   Maybe with P/T help . . .
my friendly lady-friend neighbor,

just a wall between us, always cries
when they try to give her a pill,

"Curses nurses, nurses curses,"
but she loves the Rabbi story,

loves it! Says it would make
a wonderful Bar Mitzvah speech

so I tell it again. Then we try it.
We pretend we're flamingoes,

hobbling along. *One leg each,*
two good legs between us!

Pink is also an interesting
proposition. So is flamingo.

-knock

Again?

Knock-knock, again.

Again who?

Boo-hoo.

Boo-hoo who?

Boo-hoo you.

    Nah . . .

Knock-knock

Who's there?

Like it or

Or what?

Like it or lump it?

    Nah . . .

Knock-knock.

Stop equivocating!

You know, this is getting old.

And so are you!

Knock-knock?   *Knock-knock.*

Anyone home?

Please Finish the Conversation

Welcome to the House of Uninvited Guests.
Want to try to get their attention? Get a word in?
I'm awake most of the time when they leave me

bored-to-death. Try to sleep, come evening,
all at once they're here. How many bells
did you hear? They're crowding the kitchen

around the little pot of tea. Kettle keeps whistling,
open honey jar a buzzing hive of conversation.
They never finish what they're saying. This house

gives me a headache. Again the cursing cousin.
Who let her in? And Mother instructing the mayor
on how he's supposed to remember Father.

I should have sat her down long ago, gotten
the whole story. How long could it take? Eight
hours? What's eight, or three, or eleven? Nurse!

Daughter! More numbers, green lines jumping
the overhead screen. Who ever gets the whole story,
beginning to end? Give them all the lie-detector test!

"Oh yes, and it's so good to see you . . . come in."

Hello, Mrs. Wilson

Mrs. Wilson isn't nice
and isn't mean. I've never met
anyone like that. Her toes scrunch out
a hole at the end of her shoes.
She stands by the black board
all day, except lunch. She makes us:

recite the Pledge-of-Allegiance
sing Country-t'is-of-Thee
recite the Lord's-Prayer
   (sometimes twice, she forgets
      and says—*Never enough prayer!*
      and chides—*Don't they
      say it in the Jewish church?*)
also recite Psalm 23
   (she'll leaf through the Bible
      asking which psalm the class
      would like to hear . . .
      it's always green pastures)
listen to *Announcements,*
   (who's Boy-of-the-Day,
   Girl-of-the-Day? No
   Thems-of-the-Day)
guess whose Birthday it is
   (May 23, 1958)
clean out our desks
   (flip-tops hide a lot of mess)
Cleanliness next to Godliness
   (but she smells musty)

line-up to sharpen pencils
return to desks
fold hands
now in unison, in good-citizen-voices:

We're ready Mrs. Wilson!

A Squirrel from Years Ago

It's any morning for him—quick errands
across the patio, surprised by me, stops,
sizes me up, rushes off to his acorn stash.

By a wood's edge, an ironwood uprooted--
a squall as I slept?—what more have I missed?
Its leaves have already begun to gray. The fallen

trunk is poised like a bridge angled up
touching memory—
                        another fallen tree,
long ago waiting in a boyhood's wood,
its top branches sweeping beyond the visible.
We aim it, a neighborhood crew on board
this rocket ship, departing for space zones
light-years ahead, the edge of known galaxies
beyond our neighborhoods of knowledge
launching into unimagined lifetimes . . .

            I open the backdoor like a hatch.

The squirrel, up on its haunches, quizzes me—
what are you doing here? What *am* I doing here?

            We've landed in modern times.

A Lesson for This Life?

All morning I'm humming:
the world stands on three things:
Torah, prayer, & kind acts.

Even in the Minsk shtetl
they sang it. And even in Florida,
a warm version of over-there.

How can the world stand
on three things? How about
two? Two feet, two legs.

Condense the phrases: Torah acts
& kind prayer, or, kind Torah
& prayer acts. How to sing it?

Square peg in a round hole.
Lyrics have to fit the music
or no one will remember.

Maybe it's a one-legged pillar
holding it all up. Standing on one leg
like the Rabbi and the flamingo.

A *midrash*, but I can't remember
the color-name of flamingo.
They don't have flamingoes in Minsk.

My great-grandfather is a Rabbi,
studies all day and I never met him
until last night. I thought to call him

Grandpa—but he doesn't answer.
He has three legs, counting the cane,
so maybe the song got it right.

I know who he is. In my mind
I've heard his voice, soft and pure
purling Yiddish and Hebrew.

From his face, a cascade of white beard,
beautiful curls of *peyis* he twirls and
twirls. *Zayde's* arrived. That's his name.

Blessed who comes. *Baruch ha-bah.*

What to Do with Pocket Change

is in another book. Not mine.
If there's a coin for the ferryman,
drachmas or zlotys, not two-bits.

If and when I'm just a body—
Zayde told my father who told me,
the soul returns to Blessed-

Be-His-Name with an indelible
name-tag that never washes out.
When I'm just a body, one coin

for the committee who washes me.
The other I've carried from the tray
of the *pidyon haben.* The Kohane

needed five silver pieces. Not sure
we had it. Was I redeemed? I am
still here, still counting—Doctor!

Doctor, your patient is calling.
If he's dead he'll want his eyes
closed. Or maybe, he'll want one

left open, the secret, roving one,
the sacrilegious one. Only Moses
could look into G-d's face. (Holy

Moly!) Afterwards he glowed
in divine sunburn. If and when . . .
a coin on just one eye.

(Knock-knock . . .
I don't want to miss a thing.)

Post-script: In a Nearby Park

Tap, tap,
> the jump rope snap.

Tap, tap,
> let rope slap:
>> *Birdie, birdie in the sky,*
>> *Why'd ya do that in my eye?*
>> *Birdie, birdie in the sky,*
>> *Gee, I'm glad that cows don't fly.*

Tap, tap,
> give the rope slack.
Tap, tap,
> now kick back:
>> What children know
>> They hardly show
>> And when they grow
>> They let it go.

Tap, tap,
> there's no stopping.
Tap, tap,
> the sky is dropping:
>> One, one in Purgatory.
>> Two, to the Crematory.
>> Ashes in the Lavatory,
>> Singing in the Oratory.

Tap, tap,

not to weep,

tap, tap,

if in sleep

tap,

tap,

tap,

keep,

keep

Another Post

if I keep an eye open
after life and beyond what

what might
through the orbit's pool
draining until

until the end and the op-
thamologist of sight
won't speak about
the dark
harbingers floating by,

refuses and refutes
our many colleagues
their role as tha-
natologists—
               Perhaps I heard
a sigh.
        He's still the scientist
of seeing and he knows.

I know.
"They look like worms,"
and tell him. I'm not ready,

ready for the drawling into,
into and through,

though yes
I try to get myself ready,
give myself up
to a floater being

being carried away
on a stretcher of wild blue.
The ride is gentle

into the pure and yonder,
the unclaimed

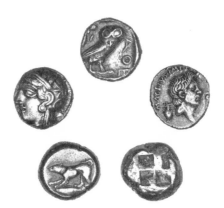

NOTES:

p 10. The unofficial song of the Civil Rights Movement of the 1950's and 60's, first composed by Rev. Charles Tindley in the gospel tradition, "I'll Overcome Someday." In 1957, Dr. Martin Luther King visited the Highlander Folk School in Tennessee. Pete Seeger played the song which he had learned at the school and taught it to the audience. Seeger recorded it in 1963. Joan Baez sang it at the 1963 March on Washington and again at Woodstock, 1969.

p 13. There are no formal "lessons" to orient an individual to a Care Home, or Nursing Home. The number is random, but alludes to the age of Bar Mitzah, 13, when "a boy becomes a man." The midrash (an instructive story) refers to a request made to Hillel (Jewish sage of the first century BCE) that he explain the entire Torah standing on one foot. Actually he did not say "Love your neighbor", but rather "Do not do to your neighbor what is hateful to you. All the rest is commentary. Now go study." He is frequently misquoted, as I have done here.

p 21. "The world stands on three things: Torah, prayer, and good acts," (*Al Shaloshah Devarim*), attributed to Rabbi Shimon, 3rd century, BCE. A song most children attending a Hebrew school are taught. *Peyis*, Yiddish for curled sideburns. *Zayde*, Yiddish for grandfather. *Baruch ha-ba* Hebrew for Blessed he who comes, a tradition welcome and a blessing said on arriving in Israel.

p 23. "The committee who washes me" references the Hevreh Kadishah, responsible for washing and sitting with the body before burial. *Pidyon haben*, a ceremony, mainly observed by Orthodox Jews, in which the first born son is redeemed from the high priest who would have a claim on him. Typically, five silver coins are given as the baby is passed around on a silver platter. The "pocket change" represents both the coins for this redemption as well as coins for the ferryman to cross the River Styx.

ACKNOWLEDGMENTS

How I Started to Use a Cane, in a slightly different version, appeared in "Southward", 13A, 2017, short listed for the Gregory O'Donoghue 2017 International Poetry Prize.

Lesson #13 from the Care Home, in a slightly different version, appeared in "Storm Brain: The Hippocrates Book of the Brain", Hippocrates Press, London, 2021.

Please Finish the Conversation appeared in "The Missouri Review", vol 42 no 1 & 2, 2014.

A Lesson for This Life? and *What to Do with Pocket Change* appeared in "Lehrhaus" (February 13, 2024).

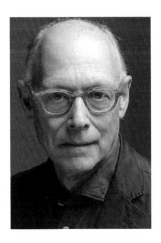

OWEN LEWIS, author of three prior collections of poetry and two chapbooks. Awards include the 2023 Guernsey International Poetry Prize, the 2023 Rumi Prize for Poetry, The Jean Pedrick Chapbook Award (*best man)* and the International Hippocrates Prize for Poetry and Medicine. *Field Light* was a "Must Read" selection of the Mass Book Awards. At Columbia University he is Professor of Psychiatry in Medical Humanities and Ethics.

Author Photo by Francesco Barasciutti

Other books by Owen Lewis
published by Dos Madres Press

Sometimes Full of Daylight (2013)
best man (2015)
Marriage Map (2017)
Field Light (2020)

He is also included in:
Realms of the Mothers:
The First Decade of Dos Madres Press - 2016

For the full Dos Madres Press catalog:
www.dosmadres.com